Rest Is Sacred

# Rest
# Is
# Sacred

Reclaiming Our Brilliance
through the Practice of
Stillness

## Octavia F. Raheem

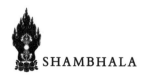

SHAMBHALA

Shambhala Publications, Inc.
2129 13th Street
Boulder, Colorado 80302
www.shambhala.com

Cover art: "Deep Into the Light" by Tracie Cheng,
www.traciecheng.com.
Cover design: Claudine Mansour

Interior design: Greta D. Sibley

9 8 7 6 5 4 3 2 1

First Edition
Printed in the United States of America

Shambhala Publications makes every effort to print
on acid-free, recycled paper.
Shambhala Publications is distributed worldwide by
Penguin Random House, Inc., and its subsidiaries.


LIBRARY OF CONGRESS CATALOGING-IN-PUBLICATION DATA
Names: Raheem, Octavia F., author.
Title: Rest is sacred: reclaiming our brilliance through the practice of stillness /
Octavia F. Raheem.
Description: First edition. | Boulder, Colorado: Shambhala, [2024]
Identifiers: LCCN 2023058045 | ISBN 9781645473275 (trade paperback)
Subjects: LCSH: Rest.
Classification: LCC BJ1499.R4 R34 2024 | DDC 204/.4—dc23/eng/20240318
LC record available at https://lccn.loc.gov/2023058045

*For my grandmamas,*

*Annie Mae Williams and Ora Faith Ramsey*

When I rest, I hear your sacred songs.

I feel your most fervent prayers.

I remember who I am. I remember whose I am.

*Opening Prayer*   xi

*Introduction*   xiii

PART ONE: Rest Is Refuge   1

PART TWO: Rest Is a Reclamation   49

PART THREE: Rest Is a Revelation   93

*Closing Prayer*   129

*Closing: Moving Forward*   131

*Acknowledgments*   133

*About the Author*   135

This is an invitation. This is a portal.

# Opening Prayer

Let us begin with a prayer.

Divine One of Rest,

You said come to me, all you who are weary and burdened, and I will give you rest. Come with me by yourselves to a quiet place and get some rest. You said I will fight for you; you need only to be still. You said be still and know.

And here we are. Here, being this portal within these pages. Here, being this place. Here, at this altar called right now.

We come in gratitude for our Ancestors who are well enough in spirit to tend to our wellness. Because of them, we found a way to rest. We made a way to rest.

We are here to reclaim rest as our birthright. Let it be so.

Let this process of reading, resting, and reflecting restore us to a natural rhythm and pace that refines our sight and bends our ears toward clarity and truth.

Divine One of Rest, we surrender to your embrace.

We are here to reclaim our brilliance through rest. Let it be so.

We may be among the first in our lineage to feel rested. To trust rest. To be safe enough to embody rest. We will not be the last.

Give us the courage to slow down, rest, and be at ease in a world that thrives and capitalizes on our exhaustion.

Soften our strength so that we may yield, again and again, to the wisdom in these pages.

A rested body is a free body. A rested heart is a liberated heart. A mind at ease is a mind that can change any paradigm.

There is power in rest. There is power in rest. There is power in rest.

When we rest, we wake up that power and ignite our brilliant potential.

And so it is.
Amen

# Introduction

Dear You,

I don't know exactly what happened that brought you here. Here to these words. Here to this book. Here to this invitation to rest. I just know it happened.

Perhaps the ground of your being and growth brought you here.

Here is a place to pause.

Take a pause.

Perhaps the deep desire to rest pointed you in the direction of the words that are now two-stepping against your heart and the book that you hold in your hands.

Your hands have been marked by time.

I don't know exactly what happened that brought you here. Here to these words. Here to this book. Here to this invitation to rest. I just know it happened.

Perhaps it was something like this.

Breathing steady, you walked down the aisle. You got married. Married to that job. You devoted your heartbeat, breath, and vitality to it. Then they asked you to leave without considering your future or plans. Or maybe you decided to go.

Your plans for birth turned into a colossal storm. In the midst of a storm, you decided it was time to change everything. And so you did it.

Everything is beautiful, amazing even. Yet still, you have an intense and unshakeable feeling something heavy is coming or someone is leaving.

After all the nightmares, your dream came true.

True, this is another threshold.

A threshold, like a half-open door. A door or an open window. A window to look through and see horizons that stretch across your eyes when you close them.

Close your eyes. See the place where the ocean and sky meet? Where they meet inside of you is a place of possibility. Possibility is the horizon and the place between two shores. Between two shores of what was and what will be—*that*.

That is what you hold in your hands. This is what you hold in your hands. You hold a companion who has been waiting for you. Precisely here. Precisely now.

After the memorial and before you can fathom how to live with your loss.

Before the breakthrough and somehow reassembling after the breakdown.

After the muscadines have fattened and fallen, and before the last trees undress.

Before the truth has been revealed and after the lie has been told.

After the sunset and before the sunrise.

This is what you hold in your hands.

A companion who has been waiting for you. One who is holding enough light for you to get your bearings and praying for you to find your way.

Close your eyes to see.

You are holding a thread to follow, a way forward.

And you are also being held.

I have been where you are.

I have been where you are, and I tell you the truth of that throughout this book because it is important that you know it. I write to you with both my feet and heart bare and as a traveler on the road *away* from exhaustion.

I write to you as one who has and continues to stumble over rocks and fall into potholes.

I write to you as one who has learned to rest where she has fallen before she gets up.

I write to you as one who has found refuge, reclamation, and revelation in rest.

I write to you as one who has been carried over, through, and across.

Open your eyes to see. You are holding a thread to follow, a way forward.

Rest and read.

I have been where you are.

You are not alone.

———

I have been a teacher of rest and stillness via restorative yoga, Yoga Nidra, and meditation since 2008. I call each class a practice, which means the actual application or use of an idea as opposed to merely theorizing or thinking about it. To me, practice is a place of concentrated focus that requires my presence more than any tendency to lean toward perfection.

Though I revere and love the formal and traditional practices I study and teach, this isn't a book to spell out instructions on exactly how to do this or that in order to rest.

Reading this book *is* a rest practice, and here's what I mean.

Do not read this book in one sitting or cover to cover. *Do you hear me?* Okay.

And if you can't resist reading it cover to cover, make sure you are relaxed or lying down when you do. Take your time if you choose that route.

Be unrushed with this book. Read it. Savor each word. Let the words work on you as you rest.

Meander through the pages like you are on a stroll through terrain that is both new and profoundly familiar—because you are.

There is poetry in this book. My personal reflections are in this book. There is even prophecy in this book.

Every sacred thread is written to weave in and out of a place that we are all indigenous to, your central core, your brilliant heart. The heart of humanity.

Take your time entering this place.

I want you to read this book one page, one line, or even just a few words at a time. In this way, you will feel both the needle and the thread, the words and your awareness, merging together in a way that creates a quilt that spans time. This slowly warms you up to the truth of a reality beyond the blanket of exhaustion that threatens to consume you.

You can hold this book to your heart, invoke the Divine of your own understanding, and ask the question, *"What words will best serve me right now?"* Then open the book and receive the insight you need.

After that, close your eyes. Perhaps rest with the words for a moment. Walk with them for the day. Share them with a family member, friend, or colleague. Let the meaning unfold as the moment spreads out in front of you.

Again, reading this book *is* a rest practice when you do it in an unhurried way.

———

This book is a place to take refuge, reclaim, and receive revelation born from rest. The practice and teaching begin the moment you pick up this book and open it. The practice has begun.

Here is my hope for you as you rest and read your way forward:

- You remember how to be with your heart, your feelings, your bigness, your smallness, your fragments, your wholeness.
- You experience the words as protective friends, covering you as you venture into a place of rest and reflection.
- You slow down enough to become aware of when you need to rest before physical signals demand that you do. Stay in your body as you read.
- You remember your natural rhythm and trust your own pace. You deserve a pace that doesn't require you to chase your breath.
- As you lay down your body, you also lay down some burdens. I see what you've been carrying, and it's heavy.
- You gather your courage to create and maintain more space in your life to rest and heal.
- You are inspired to invite people in your life to rest, and to take intentional action to create safe places for yourself and others to rest. The time for this is now.
- You can let *it* be simple. Allow *it* to be easeful.
- You reclaim your capacity to imagine and dream new ways, new worlds, and new suns.

Most of all, this is an invitation.

Soften your gaze and continue.

# PART ONE

# Rest Is Refuge

When I was six years old, I almost drowned. I was swallowed by the ravenous water and pushed into a cold, wet darkness. As I sank beyond the breath of life, I tried to scream . . . *Mama. Mama! Mama!!* Over and over and over.

At the borderland of my last breath, consciousness, and life, a hand found me. A hand pulled me up. Up to a place where there was air. Up to where I found my breath. More importantly, to me, once I opened my eyes, there she was. There she was. My mama was there. She always was. She always would be.

I believed that no matter what pulled me under, when I opened my eyes and came to, my mama, Millie Rose, would be there.

In 2021, my mama transitioned from this life. Death abruptly knocked on the door and took her away before we could answer.

A grand canyon immediately formed within me where her physical presence once lived and constantly held me together. My heart and life broke open and revealed a wide, vast, and bone-chilling river.

The year following Mama's death engulfed me and then delivered me to the gut-wrenching depths of a wild-edged river.

As I descended into the curved womb of that river, I moved beyond the reach of any hand.

That river wrapped itself, a wandering and thick ribbon, around my existence. It would not let go.

My personal journey through grief has been one of yielding to the flow and force of gravity within that river.

The pain doesn't actually get better; my capacity to withstand such a monumental loss does.

A river of grief. A river of darkness. A river of disbelief. A river of disorientation. A river of loneliness. A river of misunderstanding. An unrelenting river. A long river.

Sheer will, fighting, or brute power could not save me in the river. I could only surrender.

I had no choice other than to take refuge and surrender.

And so, I did.

Rest is a place of refuge.

Taking refuge in rest taught me:

- How to befriend my pain with honesty, care, and softness.
- That ignoring grief, individually and collectively, creates more suffering and harm.
- Healing is a nonlinear spiral and requires more than time. Time does not heal all wounds. Intention, attention, and devotion to utilizing healing tools, modalities, and practices does.
- When I disregard my hard feelings, they hold me hostage, disconnect me from my heart (and everyone in my heart), and impede my ability to give and receive real love.
- Denial of heavy emotions severely limits my access to the range of my feelings that include the lighter ones like pleasure, joy, and sweetness.
- True strength requires a tender heart. My ability to survive the river and take refuge has depended on my willingness to embody tender strength and use it in the service of my own healing.
- There is no way out. The only way through is through.

We all will have years, times, or moments in our lives when we sink into the unknown, must learn how to see in the dark and how to rest and take refuge in unlikely places and ways.

We all need refuge.

A refuge of prayers. An anointed refuge. A cosmic refuge.

A place of refuge on a journey through an immense valley filled with sharp-toothed shadows.

And in that river that was a year of devastating loss for me, I birthed a new book. Praise rained, criticism snowed, meaningful work happened. Acceptance arrived. Rejection came. Doors closed. Windows opened. I failed at some things. I achieved things that I could list and also landed on lists that might impress somebody.

The course of that river could not be changed, slowed, or controlled by any of that. I needed refuge. I would emerge to attend to my present, future, and dreams. The truth remained. Grief is heavy and exhausting. I needed rest.

Maybe you are in a place where that awareness is quickly or slowly dawning on you. The awareness that you need a place of refuge.

A place to surrender from the daily fight.

You need a place of refuge.

You need a place of rest.

Rest is the most honest place you can go and meet the Divine. It is because of this that rest is true refuge. My own journey through loss has taught me this.

I.I

Where do you start with surrender?

You don't know,

so you place your one hand into your other hand,

you sit in the dark,

you don't move.

You notice your breath.

When I teach, I often ask people to consider

*Who or what is breathing you?*

What is the breath within your breath?

So you consider who or what is breathing you,

what is the true source of your breath.

You notice the chair is holding you.

You feel the steadiness of that embrace.

You do this for one minute,

and that's one minute of refuge.

**I.2**

That's where you start.

A moment of surrender.

A walk through the labyrinth of time.

A glimpse of the center

the acceptance that this path

and journey are not linear.

It is a spiral.

Healing is not a straight line.

1.3

Find or make a way to be gentle

with your life

and self.

Find a way

to release your grip

from the handle of *always doing*.

You have pushed enough.

You have done more than enough.

Gather your strength.

Place it on the altar

in service to your softness

in service to surrender

in service to lying down.

I.4

To lie down is a power,

a place to fall apart

and be knit back together.

Come here

and be undone.

Be woven, made new.

Stop hiding in that coat

labeled *I'm too busy.*

See that you

you are a holy body.

Release the sweater of fatigue.

Be covered by supple and sturdy threads,

untangled and brilliant.

This is who you are meant to be.

1.5

You have been waiting for you

to lie down, get tucked in,

and say to yourself *that's enough for now.*

No one else in the world can say that for you.

Besides, you would not believe them.

*Soften your gaze*

*Take a full breath*

*Release your shoulders*

*again and again.*

Tell yourself what you most need to hear.

Give yourself permission to rest.

1.6

You are a fighter.

You have always fought

your way through

and if you couldn't say

you won every fight

      well,

at least you survived.

The day came

when that instinct to fight

foretold your ruin.

That day of final exhales.

The day of faint pulses.

The day of final heartbeats.

Then you knew

what you had suspected

     all along:

you can't fight your way

     through

everything.

When it comes to deeper waters

you can't fight and win

     because

there is no winning.

You have to float

to save yourself.

You can't fight and float

at the same time.

The only option is surrender.

**1.7**

You are the strong one,

  *they say.*

You know that strength has broken you.

So this time you bend.

You bend into

something soft

something vast

something that will last

something that will not break

something real

something that feels

something that both laughs and cries.

You bend

into

     the truth.

You are more than strong.

You are human.

1.8

You know what it means

to hang on by a breath

and have everyone

look at you and whisper,

*Wow, he's flying.*

You know what it means

to clutch the edge of darkness

in broad daylight

and have onlookers

say, *That's such a pretty purse.*

*They carry it well.*

You know what it means

to bear the weight of

home

family

the world

against your bones

and have them swoon,

*How amazing is her dress?*

You know it's all too much.

You need space

to exhale

to be still

to move

to live.

I.9

Food, too little and too much.

Overworking in every sense of the word.

The distorted reflection

of your own eyes at the bottom

of the wine glass, again.

Relationships that consume you

until

you find a familiar comfort in the discomfort

of your own disappearance.

You sought refuge in many places.

So have I.

Do not judge yourself

for what you did in your seeking.

What a grace to find rest when it calls you.

Say your name.

This is a way to call yourself home.

You name them. You see them.

All of the people you became to protect yourself.

The perfectionist

The fighter

The one who hides

The scared one

The overthinker

The loud one

The quiet one

The spiteful one

The unforgiving one

The mean one

The kind one

The list goes on

You start

to reclaim your wholeness—

a place of refuge.

You place your one hand

into your other hand.

You close your eyes.

You whisper *hello.*

*Welcome. I see you.*

You say your own name again and again.

Piece by piece

Part by part

One by one

You welcome your whole self home.

I.II

The more rested you become,

the more of a safe person

and place you become.

You become a living

breathing refuge

as you rest,

become more grounded

and regulated.

The more you soften your gaze,

the safer you become to yourself.

The safer you are to you,

the safer you are to others.

1.12


Trust yourself.

Not your achievements.

Not what you have done and can do.

Not your roles and responsibilities.

Trust your essence,

the cosmic dust of your marrow,

the tunnel of wind and light in your heart,

your natural rhythm that was born before time.

Trust that your innate pace is enough.

Trust your breath.

Trust your healing.

You've tried everybody else's way and pace.

It's time for you to trust your own.

1.13

The places within you

that feel unworthy

quiver in the corner

>Afraid of *not* doing.

>Afraid of *not* producing

>Afraid of saying no

Instead of pushing unworthiness further away

this time

>you hold it

>you rock it

>you listen to it

>you rest with it

then it happens.

You hustled for love for so long that

you forgot that you *been* worthy.

You remember.

You were born worthy.

I.I4

Resisting rest is resisting the Divine.

It is resisting unconditional love.

It is resisting the sacred.

It is resisting Amazing Grace.

It is resisting refuge.

What part of you wants to resist all of that?

Lovingly ask yourself,

*Why?*

1.15

You realize soon enough

rest is the mystery

and place of answers.

It is empty and full.

It is the portal

to a new

dimension of light.

Unmask the dark.

See.

1.16

When chasing your dreams

causes you to lose sleep.

When being the *Girl on Fire*

inflames your joints.

When the weight of the world

eats away at your body.

When they say, *"Sis, you look good,"*

and you know you are not well.

When the speed they applaud you for

is rushing you to your end

and you want to make it all stop.

Know that you can pause

without ending it all.

When all of this is true,

remember

rest will accept you

exactly as you are.

1.17

You start to heal.

You choose your life.

Your body shakes as you learn how to return

to your own skin and live in your bones.

You leave the rat race behind for your true path

one foot in front of the other

this time, steady and slow,

because you know

the arrival place is inside.

1.18

You finally sit down.

You close your eyes.

Tears flow.

You cover your face.

You sigh.

You say,

*I want to inhabit my life,*

*not just work in it.*

*I want to write my own story,*

*not follow someone else's script.*

You realize that what got you here

has served its purpose.

It is time to turn the page.

You wanted this change so much

that you thought you could outrun your grief.

The thing is,

it was never behind you.

It wasn't chasing you

It was within you

still

you ran until you couldn't anymore.

You kept saying it's *mind over matter*

to justify the distinct way

you pushed yourself.

When you fell down, your body said,

> *This*

> *this is what matters.*

Feel.

You found the emotions you could not outpace

waiting.

Feel.

You found an unlikely place of refuge

when you finally allowed yourself to rest and

Feel.

You found your own heart.

I.20

The truth undressed in the room,

climbed into bed and told you

exactly where to look in order to free yourself

of that toxic relationship.

That relationship.

The one always taking, never giving.

Always on the way yet never arriving.

The one that rarely answered or called.

The one where absence was a whole presence.

Rest revealed a bare truth:

You are the love you seek.

1.21

You know how to dress up exhaustion

better than most

     strumming strings

     an impeccable stage presence

the spotlight makes you glow

even more than you already do.


It pays well so you open your mouth,

begin to sing the song they want to hear.

Your voice is no longer yours.

It belongs to obligation.


Their words are razors against your tongue.

You say them anyway.

You are skilled,

smile through pain.

Everyone claps

until

one day, you don't hear them

because you are gone.

You leave the golden pedestal

and elevated stage

to enter the ground level of your real life.

Tired of standing up

you put the mic down.

You don't announce it.

You simply go,

turn the spotlight off,

and rest.

1.22

You walk in circles and wish

and pray

and worry

and call out

and wail

and beg for evidence that it will be okay,

that it all works out in the end.

No such confirmation comes

so

you stop.

Sit down on the ground

in the middle of it all

the stress

the fright

the suffering

the pit of worry

threatens to swallow you.

In the stillness you sense an embrace.

The seen and unseen holds you.

You may not know what tomorrow holds.

You just know that you are held.

1.23

Now is the time to use your strength

in service of being gentle with yourself.

Here's how:

Each morning ask yourself,

*How are you?* Listen.

Before going into your default mode

of tending to everyone else, ask yourself,

*What do I need from me?* Listen.

At least once a day,

look at yourself in the mirror

and simply say,

*I see you. I am here. I love you.*

Listen.

You wore chains of external success,

a rare metal around your neck.

Pretty lockets that kept you

striving to prove

your worth.

Until

longing for new ways,

you finally woke up

and rested.

Rest unhooked one link

then another

then another.

Rest and get free.

1.25

You picked up every stone and turned it over.

You lit every candle

said every prayer

did all of the rituals with devotion.

The cards kept telling you the same answer.

*Rest.*

Could it be that simple and obvious?

*Yes.*

1.26

You learned that integrity

is keeping your word

even if it kills you.

And it almost did.

You put your dreams on hold

to do what they asked you to do

because you said you would.

When you returned to your own dreams they were still there

*Raisins in the sun*

shards of possibility

thorns of hope

festering

sagging

a load to carry.

Under the weight

every *yes* to them

turned into a *no* to your dreams.

*Amazing Grace*, how sweet the sound

you are still breathing.

It's not too late.

You gather courage and rest.

Rest creates space.

*This is a Yes* to your dreams.

*Yes* to your dreams.

*Yes* dreams.

*Yes*.

1.27

You believed you were a burden.

Who taught you that?

And who taught him that?

And who taught her that?

And who taught them that?

*I'm a burden.*

It's only a thought,

weightless, yet cumbersome.

How can something so immaterial

be this heavy?

Can't touch the thought,

    still

it has a stronghold on you.

You've hauled it around

your entire life,

bricks in a weathering bag.

Hanging on to your mind.

The moment.

The moment you begin to question this thought

This

*I am a burden*

is the moment you also

put the bag

down.

You are not a burden.

You are a blessing.

You are a blessing.

You are a blessing.

1.28

It's me.

I'm the one

standing in the need.

*I need help.*

This is a powerful prayer.

1.29

*She said,*

Don't shout about it.

Walk slowly to a quiet place.

Make a comfortable place to lie down.

Rest there.

Them with ears

them with eyes

them with wisdom

they will hear and see.

They will know.

Why is it necessary to leave what is already gone

—again and again—

and rest in the field of right now.

Rest is so much more than lying down.

For you, the grief-stricken, it is a sanctuary to fall apart and be held.

For you, the warrior, it is a safe place to lay your sword down.

For you, the writer, it is a fountain of wisdom in your pen.

For you, the wounded, it is an anointed bandage.

For you, in the storm, it is holy shelter.

For all of our dreams, it is a blue cloud cloth.

Rest is a refuge.

# PART TWO

# Rest Is a Reclamation

Rest does not ask us to do anything or to be anyone other than who we actually are.

When you rest, the opportunity to remember yourself beyond your conditions or conditioning emerges.

> *Who were you before the world told you who you were supposed to be?*
> —Danielle LaPorte

When you rest, you remember.

When you remember, you reclaim your distinct power and possibility.

Part two is some of what I have reclaimed in rest.

Read, rest, awaken memories that transform the past, present, and future.

**2.1**

*Rest unearths the real.*

In my thirties my body said, "No more" to overworking, to exhaustion, to doing the most, and speeding ahead at all costs. If you've read the introduction to my second book, *Pause, Rest, Be: Stillness Practices for Courage in Times of Change*, you know that over a decade ago, I was hospitalized with rhabdomyolysis. It almost turned fatal. Couple that with dehydration, undernourishment, overworking, disordered eating, complete fatigue, and exhaustion; this is the imperfectly perfect storm that awakened me to my physiological need for rest.

What I didn't share in the book is that just a few weeks before that hospitalization, I fell asleep at a red light while leaving my "day job" and rushing to what, back then, I proudly called my "side hustle." I don't use the word *hustle* so freely, leisurely, or proudly anymore. The Dutch origin of the word is *hutselen*. It means "to shake, to toss." After being shaken and tossed about at the edge of burnout, I had to put that word down and in its place.

So, there I was. In the middle of the city, asleep at one of the rare places I paused back then, a red light. A blaring horn startled me and woke me up.

What I didn't write about in the book is how desperate I felt when I woke up and the light turned green, demanding that I keep going. I almost cried at that traffic light because I was so tired and felt like the only way I could stop was if I had a big, bold, red signal to tell me to. Unless there was an accident, illness, or tragedy happening, I pushed the meter on my limited capacity to rest. My worth was completely tied to my work. I was so out of touch with my own power and ability to say no to work and others that I couldn't say yes to rest. I didn't believe I had the right to change pace or rest unless I was about to fall over, so I kept dragging myself around. Exhaustion was a marker of who I was. Almost an identity, a personality trait. Defining.

Here's the thing. Even after all of that—the hospital, sleeping in traffic at a red light, and other physical indicators of my need for sleep and rest—my mind was so resistant and rebellious to the idea of rest. In other words, despite the obvious threat to my life and well-being, my mind was caught in an incessant cycle of fear of slowing down, pausing, resting, and being.

My nervous system was hijacked by lived experience and conditioning; work ten times as hard for a fraction of a chance. Blood-deep, bone-deep ancestral and past memory of life-threatening consequences for taking rest and not producing on someone else's land and time propelled my mind forward even when my body was clearly breaking down. Visceral fear of being called or seen as lazy dictated that I pushed my limits around output to try to relieve myself of that worry.

Within all of this, I became increasingly curious about the disconnect between my external and internal landscape, the disconnect between my body and mind. My body had clearly said, "Stop. No more. I am in pain and tired." Yet my mind raced, kept going, and made plans for more work and more working out. My mind wouldn't stop creating things to do even when my body said, "Shawty, I'm done."

Dr. Gail Parker's research, writing, and teaching about ethnic- and race-based stress, trauma, and injury and how restorative practices can be powerful tools to address this particular kind of trauma for us *all* gave me a portal of understanding that the wiring to work myself to the bone and resulting weariness that I carried in me was older than I was.

What if your weariness and wiring are older than you?

What if the way to be free of it is both within you and older than you as well?

What if rest is the way to truly begin that process?

On one level, resting is nourishing and feels good.

On another level, rest can be excavating.

Resting on the earth is an unearthing.

**2.2**

*Rest begins in your mind.*

I am often asked to give quick tips for squeezing rest into our lives.

Here's the thing. Rest does not fit into a bag, purse, backpack, or suitcase.

We cannot push and shove it into a place that is already packed to the brim with stuff.

Rest will not be confined to a container that we have to sit on, press down, and then forcefully zip closed (am I the only one that does this with my suitcase?).

I rarely answer the "give us a quick tip question" in the way I sense that the person asking wants.

Rest is a process. Rest requires curiosity. It demands creativity. And because many of the institutions and systems informing our lives are built on labor, even exploitation of work and labor, it requires a radical spirit and willingness to find a way to rest.

Or make one.

What I can share is that the best place to start a rest practice is first in your mind. You have to consider things like:

*What do I believe about rest? What do I believe is true about work? Who modeled work for me, and what did they show and teach me? Who modeled rest for me, and what did they show and teach me? Do I believe that my work is the most valuable thing about me? Do I believe that the greatest value of another is what they can do for me, how they perform, or what they can produce? Do I feel worthy of rest and my own care? In my family of origin or lineage, what was the consequence of resting? Where/how does the impact of that live in my physical body?*

Compassionate reflection and acceptance of your personal truth is important.

As you think, so shall you act.

You can apply a simple yet profound thought reframe. Say this to yourself multiple times a day: "I am worthy of rest." Notice how that lands in your heart. Yes, your heart.

Examining the belief structure and institutions conspiring in favor of your current fatigue, overwhelm, and/or unrested state begins to address both the individual and collective root system that is very much entangled within each of us.

So get curious about what and who informs your relationship with rest and work. Untangle yourself from the thoughts that don't serve your well-being and rested self.

Start there.

**2.3**

*You can break the spell of exhaustion.*

Rest is a basic need, and yet so many do not know how to give themselves rest.

Many don't know how to extend space for rest to others.

How can you break the spell, trance, and condition of working to the bone, perpetual overwhelm, constant fatigue, busyness, and just plain tiredness?

The process is not necessarily linear, and these steps are also useful:

- **Mindset shift.** Challenge pervasive ideas about rest and work in your own mind and the collective consciousness.
- **Slow down.** Gradually shift your pace and how you move.
- **Pause.** Become aware of natural pauses, and get creative about extending the pause when you need it.
- **Rest.** Ease into a rest practice that honors your needs and wants.
- **Share + make space.** We all are worthy of rest. Support and encourage the people around you to rest.
- **Be in integrity with yourself.** If you are a leader, facilitator, caretaker, or parent, secure your rest first. That's leading and caring with integrity.

I love Viktor E. Frankl's insight on the pause:

*Between stimulus and response there is a space (or pause).*
*In that space (or pause) is our power to choose our response.*
*In our response lies our growth and our freedom.*

The pause is:
The space between each breath. The space between each word spoken. The space between "stimulus and response."

The pause is a place of power and possibility. When you speed through the organic and naturally occurring pauses in any given moment, you diminish your ability to have an empowered response to whatever the stimulus is: your situation, a problem, the news, a new opportunity, or the person in front of you. This minimizes the possibility of delivering a response that can create space for growth and freedom. This possibility exists within the smallest of moments. You realize this once you start to really pay attention. Let's pay attention.

———

How do you currently relate to the pause?

- Do you rush to fill moments of silence with sound, noise, TV, social media, or words?
- When you are sitting at a red light or stop sign, do you reach for your phone, change the station, or find a way to do something, anything other than simply sit there?

- When someone asks you a question, do you pause, then respond, or immediately lurch into an answer?
- Do you have the ability/capacity to notice the space between the inhale and exhale?
- If you can't notice the pause for three seconds, can you rest for three minutes (or more)?

Again, I know this may seem incredibly obvious. We've been conditioned to ignore the obvious, though, so I will keep pointing it out.

When you finish reading this, will you immediately start the next "to do" or pause for a single minute, literally sixty seconds, and consider what you've read?

2.4

*Rest wakes up your brilliance.*

Who were you before the world told you who you were
supposed to be?
I encountered this question from Danielle LaPorte, years ago
during a yoga class where the teacher posed it.

I thought, are you asking me to remember childhood? To act
like the imaginings of it, the dreams of it have weight and
merit now?

I almost dismissed the question. I'm a thoughtful one though.
So, I tucked it away and came back to it later.

Now, I return to it again and again.

Who were you before the world told you who you were
supposed to be?

Wide-eyed.

Who were you before the world told you who you were
supposed to be?

Endlessly creative and wildly imaginative.

Who were you before the world told you who you were
supposed to be?

Unwilling to play by others' rules, especially when they were unfair and made no sense to little me.

Who were you before the world told you who you were supposed to be?
Curious. So curious. Always asking questions and then making up my own stories and answers.

Who were you before the world told you who you were supposed to be?
Lover of Crayola- and pastel-based art.

Who were you before the world told you who you were supposed to be?
Breakdancer. True story. Don't make me do the worm! Lol!

Who were you before the world told you who you were supposed to be?
Deep listener. Sound, expression, and word gatherer.

Who were you before the world told you who you were supposed to be?
Distilled down to the marrow of my soul, a writer.

Rest is a practice of re-membering. Of recollecting who you really are.

Before I started a rest practice, I spent decades staying so busy that I forgot who I was.

When I sat down to write my first book, *Gather*, it was a homecoming. Little Octavia rejoiced within me.

You deserve the space and opportunity to re-member and reclaim who you were before the world told you who you were supposed to be.

You are worthy of rest.

Who were you before the world told you who you were supposed to be?

Make a list. Read it aloud. Share it with someone who can hold the truth with you.

Do one thing right now that honors your brilliance because that's what we are really talking about. Waking up your brilliance each time you rest and remember who you really are.

## 2.5

*Rest your way home.*

*It's like I crossed the ocean!*

This is what my son exclaimed after he demonstrated that all of his swim lessons had sunk in. He swam from end to end in our neighborhood pool.

*I crossed the ocean.*

And that's just it. We did cross the ocean.

We come from people whose relationship with water is profoundly complicated.

It was across water that our Ancestors were trafficked and enslaved.

It was on the water that a new chapter was written.

I shared this in part one. When I was six or seven, I almost drowned. It is a vividly clear memory and remains a most unlikely baptism into the power of God's grace.

That I survived still doesn't make complete sense to me or those who witnessed what happened. Only grace does.

I crossed the ocean and didn't die, though many did. This is a reality of being a Black American:

To almost drown.

To remember what others can willingly deny and forget.

To somehow make it while carrying those memories.

Century after century. Decade after decade.

Year after year. Month after month.

Day after day. Hour upon hour.

Minute by minute. Second after second.

Breath by breath.

My son and I signed up for swimming lessons together. It was challenging, emotional, humbling, and empowering to face a fear and learn something new with my son.

We cheered each other on. We compared techniques and gave each other pointers. We had moments of sheer frustration with each other.

After many lessons, I made it halfway across the water, and there's no turning back.

I came up for air. It was then I realized I'd swam halfway across the pool. My son and our swim teacher clapped and shouted. I realized being underwater long enough to swim halfway across the pool didn't recreate visceral, bone-shocking terror in me anymore.

A wave swelled in my chest. I'd reclaimed harmony with an elemental and vital relationship, one with water. One between mother and child.

Though I am still working my way across the full length of the pool, I claim the whole reclamation for my legacy, right now.

The week after I swam halfway across the pool, my son swam all the way across.

I started the crossing by facing fear and with exceptional support.
He made his own way over the full distance with courage, confidence, and joy.

We crossed the ocean and made it back home.

The next time we were at the pool, my son ran and jumped in over and over and over again.

As I watched the freedom of his flight, landing, floating, and then swimming across the water, I thought *this. This is healing lineage. This is advancing legacy.* The water is a medium to reconnect us to our elemental nature, to freedom, to healing through joy after generations of unspeakable suffering.

My legacy is shaped by the quality of my relationships, how and what we nourish one another through.

My Ancestors were forced to sacrifice family and relation- ships on the infernal altar of exploited work and labor. I believe that even in the midst of all of that, they prayed that one day I would have a choice and that I would be awake enough to not willingly choose to continue that sacrifice. I am not building a legacy centrally defined by my work. Especially work at the expense of everything and everyone else that matters.

I don't want to be so busy striving, achieving, and working to build a legacy on those eroding boardwalks that I miss and can't attend to the profoundly worthy and revolutionary one that is ripe with possibility in my most essential relationships.

Those that cause me to reclaim something that seemed indefinitely lost.

Those born of connection and courage beyond space and time.

Ones so vast, they are an ocean's width.

Those that require real love and presence for the continual crossing.

Those that not only lead into my future, they heal my present and past.

Those that leave clear somatic signs and messages for generations to come.

Signs and messages that say *beloved, here. Here is a safe way to swim home.*

## 2.6

*Remember to rest before you need to.*

A dream about a dear friend woke me up to how much we are disconnected from rest.

In the dream, I learned that a friend was in the ICU (intensive care unit) at a hospital far away from her home after collapsing during a work trip.

I instantly rushed to be by her bedside in the dream.

When I entered the hospital room, she was sitting in the bed with the most peaceful smile on her wide-eyed face.

I ran to her, held her hands, looked her in the eyes and said *why are you smiling? You are in the hospital. In the intensive care unit no less.*

She kept smiling and said, *Don't you understand? No one can bother me here. No one can request anything from me here. My to-do list has no precedent here. Someone is going to come check my heart in a minute. Then someone else will make sure I drink water and am fed. Then someone else will check my temperature. I can rest and be intensely cared for here.*

In the dream I responded *there has to be a better way to access rest and care that doesn't include illness, injury, or some other kind of life-altering experience that forces you to finally stop and rest.*

She replied *that sounds true. I don't trust that right now, and I don't know how.*

———

After that dream, I called my friend. Through tears she said *sis, you always know. I receive this message.* We rested together right then and began to create a rest and care plan that was in harmony with her very real life.

After that I spent some time feeling the weight the dream unearthed in my heart. The weight was heavy. It was also solid gold. I thought of spaces where I have received and given *intensive care* specifically for, to, and by us. It's always next-level, divine, and life-changing.

I thought of the power of individual and collective rest.

*Intensive care.* Those words would not leave me alone.

Let's take *intensive care* out of the medical frame, and ask what would one act of *intensive and collective care* look like right now?

This message is also a vital signs check:

Are you hydrated?
How are you being nourished right now?
How is your heart?
How is your body?
How is your pulse and breath?

What do you need right now?

What do you want right now?

Do you have an intensive care plan for the week, month, season ahead?

Before you need one, create one.

2.7

*Rest is protection.*

No one is entitled to your energy, though many people might think they are.

No one is more entitled to your energy than you, and those who are your most beloved.

The world really doesn't like us when we set boundaries that protect our energy, physical, mental, emotional, and spiritual well-being.

Heck, forget the world, sometimes family and long-time friends dismiss our attempts to protect our energy as being uppity, diva-like, or extra.

Still, please protect your energy. Notice who or what feels graspy. Like they are latching on and taking slow sips of your precious energy without offering anything back. Notice whose text, calls, messages, or interactions leave you feeling energized. Notice the ones that leave you drained, confused, irritated, or constantly feeling like you have to work hard to engage with them.

Take action accordingly.

Years ago, I was training with an energy healer, and I asked her how she protected her energetic field.

I was prepared for her to share an elaborate ceremony with me. Tell me about the crystals she kept activated, placed, or wore. Describe some shield she placed around herself . . . something like that.

You know what she said?
I drink plenty of water.
I sleep at least eight hours a night.
I rest between clients and sessions.
I eat nutrient-dense food.
I take walks in nature.
I make sure to practice for myself as much as I offer practices to others.

She continued, *taking care of my physical body and making sure my body is hydrated, rested, well fed, and vital keeps my energy field strong and vice versa. It's hard to keep negative energy out when I am physically run down. So, I do the basic things that are easy to overlook when you are a super spiritual being and empath. I do them every single day, and they are my ceremony to Self. Those basic things help me to not take on other people's energy. They help me stay regulated enough to sense when more boundaries and protection are needed.*

She shared more, yet the essence was, I honor my needs and my body. This stops me from leaking energy and taking on others' energy.

As a leader in your life, you need all of your energy and a consistent way to make sure you remain clear of others' projections.

This season choose one of the following that you are NOT doing as consistently as you'd like.

Drink plenty of water.

Sleep at least eight hours a night.

Rest between clients and sessions. (For you, this may be meetings or classes.)

Eat nutrient-dense food.

Take walks in nature.

Make sure to practice for yourself as much as you offer practices to others. (For you, this may be listening to yourself as much as you listen to and hold space for family, friends, and colleagues.)

Pick one and practice it for the next seven days.

Notice the shift in your energy, and then protect that shift even more by minimizing or limiting engagement in one area or with one person that just feels extra graspy.

You know what I am talking about.

You know who I am talking about.

2.8

*Rest and reconnect to your own pace.*

Leadership is many things. It also means to set the pace. What is your natural pace? Not the one you learned. Not the condition of constant rushing. What is your natural rhythm of moving through the world?

Your natural pace likely doesn't feel too slow or too fast for you. Key words, for you, not anyone else. When you are in your natural pace, you feel grounded, easefully able, present, and clear. You can take it all in stride because you determine the stride.

If you are out of touch, reacquaint yourself to your natural pace. Like, how do you really move?

Who, if anyone, are you trying to keep up with?

There is a time and place for full-on throttle and speed—to be sure.

That also means there is a time and place for the opposite. The middle way is your natural pace.

Do you move at the speed of trust or the speed of fight? Do you move at the speed of brilliance or at the heightened speed of fear and compulsion?

Is your current pace sustainable?

How can you honor more of your natural pace in your self-leadership and leadership of others?

For today, notice the pace of your movements and seemingly simple things like eating and drinking.

For this week, notice the pace of your thoughts.

For this month, pay attention to the pace of meetings, classes, and workshops that you design and lead.

For this season, pace your sacred work by including sacred rest in your scope and sequence.

Trust that when you honor your pace, you cannot be left behind.

**2.9**

*Remember that rest, even in small shifts, counts.*

Make a list of what gets in the way of you resting. If it is a specific action, obligation, or responsibility, be sure to include any feelings and thoughts that are connected to it.

Here's an example.

**Responsibility:** *I'm in back-to-back meetings all day, every day.*
**Feeling:** Overwhelm
**Primary Thoughts:** I don't have options. I don't have time
  to rest.

Once you name the thing in the way, pause, connect to your heart, and ask yourself, "Now what is the remedy to this?" By definition remedy is a medicine, application, or treatment that relieves.

In your case, it is an application to counteract the particular angst of the ONE feeling, thought, or action that gets in the way of you resting.

Let's stay with our example.

*Back-to-back meetings. Overwhelm. I don't have options or time.*

Here's an optional remedy in doses:

Dose 1: Reframe the thought, because every action is preceded by a thought: *I find a way to make time for what matters to me. Just like I make a way for work, I make a way to rest. My rest matters.*

Dose 2: Consider something you do every day, like brush your teeth, get dressed, even look in the mirror. Commit to only doing that thing that you must do every single day AFTER you have rested. Essentially, don't get dressed until you make time to rest or be still with yourself. Even one minute of stillness counts.

I know this seems so simple. And it is. We have so much conditioning to overlook, not trust, and/or dismiss the simple.

Dose 3: Start every meeting you lead with one to three minutes of rest via stillness, intentional breathing, or simply inviting others to get comfortable and take care of themselves. The smallest shifts add up.

Dose 4: Celebrate after you rest. This could simply be saying to yourself, "I see you. You did it," with a smile. This activates the reward center in your brain and creates what I am going to nonscientifically call a "delight/pleasure" imprint in your brain, making it more desirable for you to do it again.

Dose 5: Repeat the above every day.

Conscious intention and attention are required to shift anything. For you, work has been the central axis around which so much has necessarily spun.

You can acknowledge that and also make a bold choice every day to engage with yourself in a way that moves rest, your well-being, and care away from the margins and into a balanced place toward the central axis one choice at a time.

It's time to make room for your rest within your work.

Your work must make room for your rest.

One thought at a time.

Start one dose at a time.

One day at a time.
One practice at a time.

2.10

*Let the Divine do their work.*

One of my favorite grounding instructions for a meditation practice is one I heard from Lama Rod Owens, *let the chair do the work of the chair.*

Another layer to this instruction was shared with me by Executive Leadership Coach Cherese Brauer. She said, *As I get clearer and clearer on what is mine to do and what is God's to do, I have more ease and space to rest. Come to find out, I was out there pushing, dragging, and pulling—forcing life—left no room for divine support or intervention.*

In other words, let the Divine do the work that only they can do. This frees you to do yours. This frees you to dream, rest, expand, deepen, grow, and write new narratives brimming with grace.

This frees you to remember that your true destiny, as Octavia E. Butler reminds us, is *to take root among the stars.* And grow up from there.

Consider where an unseen yet felt hand is reaching and stretching toward you.

Can you sense it? Can you feel it?

This is an invitation to remember the wide cosmic embrace, yearning to hold you.

This is an invitation to ask for divine support, receive, and allow it.

Do not stay so busy doing that you forget to be.
That you forget how to be loved by the most Divine.
To be loved by the most sacred.

**2.11**

*There is rest for the weary.*

She got in my face.

I recently had someone try to shame me for talking and teaching about rest.

Or to be clearer, she told me I was misguiding people and also implied that I could be "further" along in my work, marriage, and mothering if I didn't spend so much time resting.

I listened. Took in her words.

It was a sister, a woman I consider my longest and closest friend. Within her critique, dismissal, and resistance to my devotion to rest, I heard her exhaustion, pain, and confusion. I understood it well, too well.

I heard her real concerns around financial stress and the need to always be hustling to make ends meet. I felt every word she said about having to be four times as good for half the chances.

Through sobs and tears, she yelled at me, "No one will help me get all of this shit done if I sit around daydreaming and resting!"

I heard her fear of "Who will I be if I stop defining myself through my work, performance, hyperproduction, and insatiable need to prove my worth? And what if they call me lazy? Lazy is a stigma for women like me."

Her vulnerability and pain convicted me. I began to list my

accomplishments to try to convince her of how much rest allowed me to do. I said, "Look, I opened a yoga studio within six months of giving birth to my son. "

She responded, "Yeah, and where is that studio today?"

Whew. Dang. She came with the gut punch because she knew I'd made the challenging decision to close that business in 2020. Against my best judgment, I continued to try to convince her of the power, wisdom, and necessity of rest by saying, "I've done so much in the last few years"—and listed out all of the things.

**Her:** Arms folded. Lips tight. Eyes rolled.

She was not moved. I also had a sinking feeling. Why was I trying to prove something about rest by only talking about work?

She looked disgusted, restless, and impatient as I continued to list, name drop, and try to show her how productive my rest had been in the last few years.

Tired of listing off achievements that were accelerated by my rest versus slowed down by it, I finally paused. Looked up and saw that she was shaky and her eyes were weighted with worry, sadness, rejection, and even rage.

Then I looked at her. With tears staining her face, she whispered, "And what if all of that is still not enough and you out here resting and wasting time. There is just too much to do and too much at stake and you are telling me to rest."

I looked closer. There was a mirror. This woman was me. Literally, me.

It was me. Shaming me. Criticizing my ~~work~~ purpose. Feeling the inner constraints of systemic and external oppression—including racism, sexism, and even regionalism. It was me questioning the value of rest in a world that is unjust and quite frankly on fire.

*exhale

When I move beyond the surface of the reflection in the mirror, I remember what is true.

Rest is a superpower.

I reclaim my brilliance. I have an inner knowing that the way things have been for women like me is not the way that they have to be.

I trust that another way and another world is possible.

I have faith that a well-rested woman is an unstoppable cosmic force.

I declare that my Ancestors didn't work to death and have their labor exploited for me do the same and teach that to my son as his only option or legacy.

The frantic loop of grind culture and past generational traumas that tell me that there is "no rest for the weary" is a trap. I return to my devotion to rest, to stillness, to quiet, to space, to restorative yoga and Yoga Nidra daily to get free.

Challenging and changing the long-held narrative that working myself to the bone is the only way has required commitment, beloved community to hold me accountable, honesty, and radical personal truth-telling.

Inhale.

Remember.

**Me: *rips up old script, throws it out of window. Lets afro out, dances, then goes to lie down.**

Another way is possible.

Sis, looking in the mirror. Come, rest, and wake up to your brilliance.

**2.12**

*The earth is trying to tell us to rest.*

The soil that plans to yield a great harvest for seasons and generations to come can't always be producing. At times, it must lie fallow, unsown, unseeded. It must have moments, if not seasons, where it is not being plowed, picked at, worked, or produced upon. It must rest.

Fallowing soil is a method of sustainable land management that has been used by wise farmers all over the world. On the surface such periods may look like nothing at all is happening. Yet beneath the surface, in the brilliant dark of blackness, an entire universe and ecosystem is transforming into a place that yields wild abundance.

The benefits of allowing land to lie fallow are not unlike the benefits of allowing yourself to rest.

Rest:

Increases your capacity
Provides access to dense nourishment
Offers guidance for sustainable restructuring and organizing
    toward more abundance, not less.
Yields future abundance

It's not always easy to step out of the tilling space of your work, especially in this climate and at this time.

Yet earth wisdom tells us that rest is not a luxury. It is necessary. The alternative is to completely deplete the soil, leaving your future and the next generations a guarantee of famine.

Your seeds deserve the richest soil. Our seeds deserve the richest soil possible.

The land and the most sustainable land practices teach us that devoting ourselves to periods of rest allows for the soil to become as well as possible.

We know the quality of the soil dictates the destiny of the seed.

The seedling of your dreams deserves abundant nourishment, and this requires rest.

Instead of reproducing the same old nightmares, rest creates room for new futures and dreams to grow.

2.13

*Rest and you will grow.*

It was a spring day. I heard a hum in my yard. Then, I saw one or two of my rosebuds wake up.

Rest is an essential and often missing component of sustainable growth.

Ask the rosebuds that retreat each year and gloriously expand out and upward in spring.

Humans are not rosebuds, yet we are here to take deep root, thrive, and endure beyond our season of planting.

We are here to bloom into our most brilliant purpose and expression of being.

We deserve to unfold in our glory and with ease.

Do you hear it? The sacred whisper of roses saying *we are evidence and lasting proof that true growth and longevity requires rest.*

Do your visions and goals include rest?
Does your career, business growth, or scaling process include real rest?

Do you expect the stem of your body and mind to just keep producing without ever entering into the profound nourishment of a dormant space?

Rest and you will grow.

**2.14**

*Rest reveals wisdom like:*

1. Gentle fierceness is required to maintain devotion to rest.
2. Rest can swiftly bring you to a place of clarity.
3. Is resisting rest also resisting clarity?
4. Declutter a little bit at a time and make space.
5. "Doing it all" at once overwhelms the system. Shutdown ensues.
6. Perfection isn't required. Self-honesty and presence is.
7. Don't add anything to your "to-do" list for one week. See what happens.
8. Can you get curious about what gifts your devotion and practice really want to give you?
9. Are you afraid of commitment to yourself? If so, hold that with tenderness and ask yourself why.
10. Prioritizing our truths: peace, ease, clarity, connection, agency, space . . . in a practical way requires action.
11. Eliminate autoresponse "yes." The road to freedom is paved with many a "hell nah's." Ask Harriet.
12. It feels good to move from theory, rumination, and overthinking to embodiment and mindful action that supports more rest in your life and the world.
13. It can also feel scary because it signifies that you really finna shift some stuff up.

14. An essential point of the growth process of any seed takes place in the dark.

15. What do you want to be true one year from now?

16. What are you willing to NOT do in order for that to be true?

17. What one thing are you willing to do every day to make it true?

18. Practice makes it possible.

19. Being witnessed activates deep(er) healing.

20. Jon Kabat-Zinn defines healing as "coming to terms with things as they are."

21. Bearing witness is an offer of acceptance.

22. What have you witnessed as you have read or shared these words?

23. What if it is actually easy and we have been conditioned to believe otherwise and orient toward hard?

24. Whether it's 40 days, 3 days, or 365 days—it's really one practice/one day at a time.

25. Silence is a messenger.

26. I don't have to have an answer.

27. Another word for "second-guessing" is *self-doubt*. Who planted that seed of doubt? What waters it? Eliminate whatever nourishes the doubt and second-guessing.

28. Boundaries keep you in integrity.

29. As you evolve, your idea of achievement and success gets to evolve. That's okay.

30. What does knowing feel like in your body? Follow that sensation instead of following the train of doubts.

31. You are brilliant.

32. Rest and reclaim all that you are.

## 2.15

*"No weapon formed against thee shall prosper."*

I come from a place where "no weapon formed against thee shall prosper" is not only a scripture (Isaiah 54:17 NIV). It's an initiatory mantra. It is often recited at thresholds, in the valley, at the edge, and on the mountaintop. It is offered in both peace and war, always with courage and conviction. Amid the darkness of systemic oppression, weaponizing of race, gender, class, orientation, religious expression—all the things, these words "no weapon" are a compass, light, and portal to memory.

It's a mainline of communication to my most recent and closest Ancestors.

It reminds me that the ones hoarding and wielding the biggest weapons are destined to be defeated on the ground and in the cosmos.

It invites me to consider what it means to prosper and how to win without causing cyclical harm.

I also say this often.

I am from a place where "find a way or make one" is an entire sermon of faith, a battle cry, a prayer, a call to action, an invitation to subvert, and a victory song.

These words remind me to imagine, dream, sense, conjure, create, and align my steps toward possibility where many see none.

As a Black Woman born and raised in the American South, wayfinding is in my breath, blood, and bones.

I am not the only one with this sacred thread of way making woven into the fiber of my being.

You have it too.

You have risen in the face of all manner of weapons formed against you.

You have found and made a way to survive, live, thrive, vision, dream, and redefine how to prosper for yourself, community, and honestly on behalf of us all.

This is no small thing. It's a transformative thing.

You know how to find a way or make one.

I do too.

It's in our marrow.

It's in every cell.

The map on your skin.

Now is the time to use **your** way-making power to find a way or make a way to rest.

Now is the time to use **our** way-making power to find a way or make a way to rest.

Your life depends on it. Our lives depend on it.

# PART THREE

# Rest Is a Revelation

I have done plenty of work that I am truly proud of, and every day that I wake up and rest with a leader, I literally shout GLORY!

The world needs more well-rested leaders who have internalized what it means to move at the speed of trust.

A while back, I had a dream that felt so real, I could smell the well-seasoned earth in it when I woke up.

In the dream many people were walking through a field of wildflowers carrying baskets and blankets.

At the front of the line, there were elders who walked with pure grace and dignity.

Behind them, there were people of all ages who strolled with ease, lightness, and an air of vitality and joy.

Behind them, there were teens, children, toddlers, and wobbly little ones who moved freely, giggled, jumped, danced, skipped, and played along.

Behind that, there was a Great Divine Parent and Guardian whose presence felt protective. They were the keeper of the processional. They held the littlest ones and elders who couldn't walk on their own in their vast embrace.

I was in that line as my current self. My future self stood with outstretched arms and head tilted toward the sky in the middle of the field as a witness to the generations of well-rested people gathering for a rest reunion.

My Ancestors and descendants were represented in every layer of the line. Forward and back.

The line slowly turned into a circle. Everyone put down their baskets, spread out their blankets, and laid down in a clearing under a quilt of gold-laced blue sky in the warm sun.

The Great Parent placed the babies and eldest of elders down and began to hum a lullaby full of wisdom, prayers, and incantations to set us free from the bondage of overworking.

Everyone began to hum. The ground, trees, birds, and butterflies did too.
Then, there was a collective inhale followed by an exhale.

After that, we rested in complete silence.

I woke up with tears in my eyes. I felt a wave of peace, healing, clarity, and purpose.

It was all a dream. It was also real.

Rest is a revelation.

Rest reveals what is possible and clears our eyes. Rest can show us a new vision and release us from the tyranny of *how* it will all unfold. There is a part of us that already knows. That part is often covered in thick tapestries of exhaustion. The blanket of rest dissolves the parts of us that continue to align with collective confusion and amnesia instead of remembrance and clarity.

So much revelation is waiting for us to slow down, untangle from the frayed fabric of compulsive busyness, and finally listen.

3.1

Every Ancestor you have is alive
in your body right now.
Every descendent that will be
is in your body right now.

Rest heals your past, present, and future.

Gather your granddaddy's blankets
Let them cover your dreams.
Go and get your great grandmama's quilted pillows
Place them under your knees.

Your rest rewrites their history,
creating an ancient beginning

Rest and give birth to new endings.

## 3.2

This is a place to put old bones down
to reset and restructure
resurrect
starlight
red clay
sand
your body.

This is a place where hearts
and minds follow breath
through portals to reach
galaxies of quiet.

There is no performance to render.
The most productive thing to do
is nothing
      except
witness what rises up within you
when you lie down.

Whatever comes up when you rest
comes to be healed.

3.3

You planted seeds that bloomed in the sky.

When you rest
you can look up
and see the course
charted before you had a name
before you had a body
and definitely before you had a job

This is what saves you from being crushed in the grind.

You live close enough to the ground
that when you gaze up
you see a map.

The map has a full view of the way.

Your future is planted in the stars.

3.4

Presence is greater than perfection.
Presence is greater than performance.
Presence is greater than pretending.

You
your family
your friends
your community
our world

We do not need any more
pretending
solely performance-driven
perfectionism.

We need presence
to see what actually is
and create what can become.

3.5

If your true destiny
as Octavia E. Butler reminds us
is to *take root among the stars*
and grow up from there
you'll need to know
how to expand
across time
reach new heights.

The answer isn't found
in more work
The answer is
right there.
It is tucked in a fold
in your imagination.

3.6

You are an embodied example of how to breathe with your whole life.

You teach the children and elders how to live and no longer fear their own deep breaths.

You love so completely that in your presence, everyone feels real love.

You share yourself without depleting yourself.

You are a safe place to be.

This.

This is the new measure of prosperity in this new era.

3.7

One day you woke up, and you proclaimed it.

This is Day One.

Not one day.

~~One day I'll start.~~

~~One day I'll stop.~~

~~One day I'll rest.~~

~~One day I'll write.~~

~~One day I'll wake up.~~

~~One day I'll say no.~~

~~One day I'll say yes to.~~

~~One day I'll trust.~~

~~One day I'll leave.~~

~~One day I'll return.~~

~~One day I'll dance.~~

~~One day I'll celebrate.~~

~~One day I'll . . .~~

Not one day.

Today is Day One.

Day One of remembering your brilliance.

This is day one of resting without apology.

3.8

You are a child of the Divine.
A flower of the Universe
uncontained

Free.

When you live from that wisdom
you release the fragrance of truth,
an earthen musk,
hints of old redwoods
in the room.

When you walk in that truth
you leave the scent of luminosity,
newborn skin,
drops of liquid gold,
and suns rising
in every space that you enter.

Your aroma lights up the whole world.

3.9

You left it all behind.
It was worth it.
You are worth the effort it takes
to rest, dream, remember, and become.
You are worth the time it takes
to reconnect to your imagination
in a world that sells prepackaged dreams.

Imagination is a power.
Imagination is a power
that you recollect in rest.
And
You did it.
You danced away from those doors,
ladders, and ceilings of "opportunity."

You found a doorway to untapped potential.

Now, the sky is your floor.

There is no limit.

3.10

There is magic in your hands.
Enough to change the ending.
Rewrite the beginning.

The way it has been is not the way it has to be.

In fact,
the moment you take your hands off the machine
and relieve them of the grind
is the moment your fingertips begin to shimmer and sing.

You remembered.
You remembered
your hands belong to you,
not endless labor.

This transforms your story.

This frees your hands to deliver.

Your magic returns to you.

3.11

Your body holds more than your own stories.
It holds the lamentations and praise of those who came before you.
It holds the laughter, utterances, and tears of those yet to come.
Every word is a hymnal that echoes through the hallway of time,
*I am here. I am here. I am here.*

3.12

She asked, *What will be different because you were here?*
She replied:
*People breathe easier because I was here.*
*People laugh more because I was here.*
*People have greater access to their tears because I was here.*
*People are more gentle with themselves, each other, and the earth because*
*I was here.*

3.13

It's all holy ground.

Everywhere you stand is holy ground.

Treat it as such.

Everyone you meet is a sacred place.

Everyone.

Treat them as such.

The past, present, and future

are always co-creating one another on holy ground.

Remember that.

3.14

The earth is soft, heavy, and generous again.

Green-kissed mountains stand at the gate of heaven and pass time with the clouds.

At dusk, you sit on the edge of a circular porch and listen to the sound of one hundred thousand raindrops falling to their destinies.

They are so easy, grace-filled, and free in their letting go.

You want to be like them, so you study them.

Let the raindrops become your teacher.

3.15

Here, you can walk on red dirt
and still touch the sky,
between starshine and clay.

The air weaves together
a thick blanket of peace,
and you rest your plans and worries.

You recollect who you are
and whose you are.

Before Civil Rights
jim crow,
and reconstruction.

Before bondage
crossing the wide ocean
the Door of No Return.

Now, no longer bound,
no more chains holding.
Holding your mind in a fixed state

Rest unlocks the healing
the medicine
the wisdom that is in your lineage.

Rest is the key to set you free.

3.16

An Ancestor dreamed you here
to end the cycle of overwork, exhaustion,
and depletion in your lineage.

Somebody prayed you here
for healing on an individual
and collective level.

Look up
It is written in the sky

This time you get to heal through joy.

3.17

You rest and heal your fear that if you don't do everything on the ever-growing checklist you won't be worthy of love.

You rest and rediscover a tender place in your own heart.

Then you are touched by life.

Then you touch life with a lighter hand.

3.18

You start each day with reverence for life and breath.
You write love notes to yourself
instead of making never-ending "to-do" lists.

Now

You acknowledge your heart.
You tune in to your body and breath.
You write prayers to unfold
blessings throughout the day.

3.19

You define success by:
How often you are present to the beauty and awe around you
How often you smile when the moon rises and wakes up in the
evening
How often you stop to delight in the sun kissing your neck

Success is when you remember
there are infinite possibilities available to you
because you slow down enough
to see the evidence
in a million shades of green
gracing the earth.

3.20

You trade in the urgent life
for a softer one
that includes rest on the green belly of the earth

sky gazing.

You almost missed this
sweet life in pursuit of
someone else's idea
of what you should be and do.

You know you aren't the only one
who is worthy of this kind of life,
so you create space for others to rest.

Space ripples through all of your relationships,
makes deeper connection
Your love grows as you rest and become

become more fulfilled from the inside out.

3.21

When you offer yourself
less harm
less judgment
less criticism
less blame
more grace
more kindness
more tenderness
more care
more healing
you are able to extend that to others.

Then
You move at the speed of life.
Then you move at the speed of truth.
You move at the speed of sacred love.

3.22

It seems simple.
Yet so many have completely lost their way.
What does it mean to move at the speed of life?
A twenty-four-hour period has both day, night, dawn, and dusk.
An orchestra of heat from the sun.
A symphony of quiet from the moon.
Of course there are stretches of time
that require working, doing, and movement.

That also means there are transitions
in between all of it that deserve
slowing down, stillness and reflection.

Remembering this is a revelation.
Refuse to forget it.
Find your way.

3.23

When you move at the speed of life,

It's free of the anxiety of giving or receiving an immediate response.

You encourage others to rest.

You don't talk about it. You are about it.

You know how to honor that there's a season for all things.

There's a time for all things, not just work.

There's a time for all things, this includes rest.

3.24


S l o w

Intentional

Steady

We dismantle disordered systems from within

The weight of oppression is real

And the truth is

It is not mine

It is not yours

It is not ours to carry any further


We have carried enough
Too much, in fact

We are done.

We will rest and be free

We will wake up and walk forward
Lighter
Together

3.25

We gathered our energy when we rested.
With new energy,
whole, and intact,
we ended our entanglement with disordered systems.

We ended our dysfunctional relationship with
the ones that told us we were
the producer and the product.
The ones that made our Ancestors
forced free labor.
The ones that taught us that our only value
was in our work.

The same ones that treat
Others' disposal
like throwaways
and devalues our lives
and even our deaths.

The ones that will not accept our *nos*,
coerce us into *yes*,
and then deny any fault
in the suffering or injury that follows.

The ones
that dismiss our boundaries
and refuse to affirm the brilliance
of our continued existence despite it all.

S l o w
Intentional
Steady
We dismantle all of that.

We orient toward our innate rhythm.

Slow
Intentional

We receive the revelation
the memory
That we are sacred.
That we are brilliant.
That we are unbroken.
All of us.

3.26

When you rest, you ease
ease the pressure in your blood
and on your heart.
The pain in your back
the contraction and heaviness
in your pelvis, hips, and shoulders
the throbbing in your head, feet, and hands
All of that eases.

May ease become your legacy.

May you pass it on to your descendants.

3.27

You include others in your rest.

You gather with people you love and rest.

You congratulate people on *doing nothing*.

You create schedules that include rest.


You are free of the trance of fatigue and busyness.
You free others from the spell of always grinding.

Your wholeness isn't derived from what's on your calendar.
It comes from within and from the time you spend
In presence
in nature
in connection
in truth
in sacred space.
In love
And
with others.

3.28

The future belongs to the well rested.
To those who are committed to presence more than performance.
The well rested are not those who shrink from accountability and responsibility.

In fact, the well rested are the opposite.

They are the ones who understand that
the only way to fully wake up their dormant power is through rest.

They understand that the movements of the future will
be imagined, discerned, and revealed to them in quiet and stillness.

The way forward will only be revealed
from your most rested and awakened heart.

The collective way forward will only be revealed
from our most rested and awakened heart.

Pause and listen.

3.29

They no longer ask, *What do you do?*

They inquire and share:

What are you here to heal within your lineage?

What are you here to rest or relieve within your lineage?

What does your work allow you to heal within you?

What does your work heal in the world?

What part of you is allowed to rest or access relief through your work?

What does your rest heal within you? The world?

3.30


It is all a dream.
It can also become real.
I rest and wake up.
You rest, and you wake up.
The more people rest,
the more people wake up
to brilliant possibilities and
ways of being.

This is how we save ourselves.
This is how we save each other.


We rest.

# Closing Prayer

Divine One of Rest,

Thank you for revealing the truth that Rest is Sacred.
Thank you for the refuge, reclamation, and revelation written
in these pages. Thank you for your presence and for being a
soft place to land.

As we go forward, let us remember that rest is the bridge between where we are and where we want to be.

Rest is home.
Rest is a channel to memory.
Rest is a doorway to our hearts and the heart of humanity.

Rest is sacred work and deserves devotion.

Bind any and all distractions that try to get in the way of our rest.
May no weapon formed against our rest prosper.

When rest calls, let us have the courage, clarity, and wisdom to answer the first time.

May our rest wake us up to the brilliant power of simply being.

And so, it is.
Amen.

# Closing

*Moving Forward*

We are at a critical moment in our collective history. The world is on fire, and here I am writing about rest and inviting you to rest. While writing I wondered if you'd think, *She's calling me into a burning house and telling me to lay down?*

True. There's a fire. Have you slowed down enough to ask who and what tends to the insufferable fire, expanding its reach and devastating impact? What systems, conditions, and repetitive patterns feed the monstrous blaze? And what starves it?

These questions were my companions as I wrote the prayers, poems, and reflections in this book.

Rest is Sacred, yet is it enough for where you are right now? Is it enough for where we collectively are right now? Is it the holy water we need to extinguish the fire?

Here's what I know.

Rest is a start. It is an invitation to get out of the burning house before it or we completely collapse. It is the soothing siren to wake up before it all falls down.

It is a portal to envision a gateway to safe harbor.

Most of all, I know that rest is a healing salve with brilliant regenerative power. And we need that kind of anointed power right now.

# Acknowledgments

Thank you:

Divine One of Rest

Ancestors

Red Clay

Starshine

Beloveds

Teachers

Students

Sisters

Friends

Devotees

Dream Keepers

You know who you are

&

I am because you are.

# About the Author

Octavia F. Raheem is a wife, mother, author, rest coach, and restorative + Yoga Nidra teacher. She is the founder of Devoted to Rest®, a transformational rest-focused immersion for visionary leaders making a high impact in their fields. She teaches passionate and driven individuals how to awaken their fullest potential through the power of rest. With 10,000+ hours of training and teaching experience, she is a true luminary in the areas of rest, restorative arts, wellness, and yoga. Octavia has been featured in the *New York Times*, *Yoga Journal*, *Well+Good*, *Tricycle*, at Essence Festival (Atlanta), and more.